THE
✚DANIEL
PLAN

JUMPSTART GUIDE

DAILY STEPS *to a*
HEALTHIER LIFE

FAITH + FOOD + FITNESS + FOCUS + FRIENDS

RICK WARREN D.MIN.
DANIEL AMEN M.D.
MARK HYMAN M.D.

≣ ZONDERVAN®

P9-CEC-442

ZONDERVAN

The Daniel Plan Jumpstart Guide
Copyright © 2014 by The Daniel Plan

This title is also available as a Zondervan ebook.
Visit www.zondervan.com/ebooks.

Requests for information should be addressed to:
Zondervan, 3900 Sparks Dr SE Grand Rapids, Michigan 49546

ISBN 978-0-310-34165-9

Interior design: Sarah Johnson
Interior illustration: Sarah Johnson

Printed in the United States of America

18 19 20 21 22 /DPM/ 22 21 20 19 18 17 16 15 14 13 12 11 10 9 8 7 6 5 4

God's Prescription for Your Health

Welcome to The Daniel Plan. We are glad you picked up this 40-day guide. It's designed to help you jumpstart your journey to health. You will be introduced to The Daniel Plan Essentials: Faith, Food, Fitness, Focus, and Friends, which are the foundation for getting healthy in every area of your life.

Thousands of people have now experienced the life-changing benefits of The Daniel Plan lifestyle. We have been inundated with stories of transformation. Not only do participants feel better, but they are also able to finally lose weight, keep it off, and discover greater energy and better sleep. The Daniel Plan lifestyle has allowed many participants to get off medications and minimize chronic illnesses. We have asked them how the program worked best for them and what principles were key to their success. This guide reflects their answers: the proven, real-life tools and resources that will help you reclaim your health.

You will learn to rely on God's power instead of your own willpower. Each day will provide biblical inspiration and practical tips and tools to help you make progress one step at a time. This journey is all about grace and peace. The goal is progress, not perfection.

As you begin to eat foods that love you back, you will start to feel better and you will be motivated to explore new foods and recipes that will infuse nutrition and goodness into your body and mind. You will discover movement you enjoy, and you will recognize that The Daniel Plan lifestyle is rooted in abundance, not deprivation. You will live out Romans 12:2 as you are renewed by the transforming of your mind.

This is not a journey to do alone. In fact, we encourage you to invite at least one friend to join you for support and encouragement, which you need to stay the course. We have discovered that friends are the secret sauce of The Daniel Plan. Every *body* needs a *buddy*.

Each day we will walk you through key principles related to faith, food, focus, or friends. For fitness, we will point you to our existing 40-day Fitness Plan in the book *The Daniel Plan: 40 Days to a Healthier Life* and check in with you throughout the week to monitor your progress.

Every ten days has a main focus to set you up for success and give you a vision for what's coming. Then at the end of every 10 days, we will remind you to pause, celebrate, and recalibrate. This will give you a chance to celebrate your motivations, victories, and changes. You will also examine challenges and shift your perspective, so rather than viewing them as failures, you see them as opportunities.

We all have a different starting point on the journey toward better health. This guide gives you guidance and options so that this plan is yours. You design it based on your preferences and the pace you want to set for yourself. If you want an early win and want to set the stage for fast results, we highly encourage you to do the 10-Day Detox. We will tell you more about that on Day 9. If you decide you would rather take it slowly, your long-term success will ultimately depend on integrating the five Essentials of Faith, Food, Fitness, Focus, and Friends into your everyday life.

The Five Essentials

Each of us is in a different place with our health, but the Essentials — Faith, Food, Fitness, Focus, and Friends — will hold up your life, enliven your body, enrich your mind, and fill your heart.

FAITH

Health comes from recognizing and using God's power in your life and treating your body and mind with the care that he intended. When you learn to rely on God's power, you have the key to lasting change. Spiritual health gives you a foundation for building habits and perspectives for health in any area.

FOOD

You can actually eat anything based on one rule: Eat real, whole food. Eat a colorful variety of real, whole foods from real ingredients that you can make yourself — or that are made by another human nearby. If it was grown on a plant, eat it. If it was made in a plant, leave it on the shelf.

Simple, real, fresh, delicious, nutrient-packed foods that are easy to cook, foods that come from a farmer's field not a factory, foods that traveled the shortest distance from the field to your fork — that is what we should eat. A chicken, a vegetable, a bean, a nut, a grain, a fruit, an egg. Everything else is fake food that depletes energy and health. Real food heals and nourishes. So eat real, whole foods made by God.

FITNESS

Your body is designed to move and become Daniel Strong. What images come to mind when you think of the word *strong*? Do you think of the prophet Daniel? Daniel possessed strength that went well beyond the size of his muscles.

Daniel Strong = A pursuit of excellence in body, mind, and spirit for God's glory.

Before you even start a fitness plan, the key to success is to choose activities you enjoy doing.

Take the Daniel Strong Challenge to improve your fitness, combining prayerful movements, loosening breaks, active games and aerobic activity, and youthful strength training into your life, and watch what happens! We encourage you to do the fitness challenge for 40 days to change your fitness habits. To begin — even if you have never exercised regularly or haven't in a long time — go to chapter 9 in

The Daniel Plan Book, where you will receive a "play of the day" and a plan that focuses on all the aspects of fitness you have just learned — in small, doable steps.

FOCUS

You can have solid faith, healthy food choices, and plenty of exercise and still sabotage your health. The potential saboteur? Your brain. When your brain works right, you tend to be happier, physically healthier, and more thoughtful, because you make better decisions.

Two of the most important parts of the Focus Essential are to know your motivation and renew your mind. This requires disciplining your mind to have accurate, honest thoughts and bringing your attention each day to those things each day for which you are grateful.

FRIENDS

When it comes to your health, every *body* needs a buddy. We need each other. In fact, the New Testament says over and over to love one another, encourage one another, serve one another, support one another.

Research shows that people getting healthy together lose twice as much weight as those who do it alone. Friends are the secret sauce of The Daniel Plan.

TODAY'S STEPS

1. Assess your health in each of the five Essentials before you start and again at the completion of the program. Go to *danielplan.com/start* and click on the link for "Essentials Survey."

2. Start reading *The Daniel Plan: 40 Days to a Healthier Life.*

3. Begin The Daniel Plan 40-Day Fitness Challenge; see chapter 9 of *The Daniel Plan* book.

Know Your Motivation

Commit everything you do to the LORD. Trust him,
and he will help you. (Psalm 37:5 NLT)

One of the most important parts of the Focus
Essential is to know *why* you want to get
healthy. Without a clear sense of motivation, it is
harder to stay the course. But once you know why
you care and must be healthy, your motivation fuels
you to stay focused. Ask why you want to be healthy.
Is it to live in God's will? To have mental clarity? Or
to be a great role model for someone you love?

Write down your motivation — and look at it daily.
It's most effective if you approach it from two perspectives: To attain benefits and avoid consequences.

For example, participant Mandy Cameron told
us, "My greatest motivation is to model the Lord for
my grandchildren and to work with children.... I
notice the responses of others when I look good and
feel good; I even notice the nudgings of the Lord
more clearly. Perhaps this relates to having a sense of
contentment and well-being. I am more loving and

more compassionate when my body temple is functioning closer to optimum operating level."

Write what you believe God wants for you and what you want for yourself in each of the Essentials. Use the results from the Essentials Survey to guide you. Be positive and use the first person. Write your purpose with the expectation that with God's power it can happen. If you need to, work on it over several days. After you finish with the initial draft (you will frequently want to update it), place this list where you can see it every day, such as on your refrigerator, in your phone, or as your desktop wallpaper.

Fitness: Another important piece that will help you make progress is your health numbers. Find out and record your basics: height, weight, BMI, blood pressure, waist measurement, hips measurement, and activity level (sedentary, light, regular, active, vigorous). *The Daniel Plan Journal* includes pages to record these numbers, or you can star your free Health Profile online *danielplan.com/start/*.

TODAY'S STEPS
1. Write down your motivation for better health. Post it where you can see it every day.
2. Know your health numbers.

Commit Your Plans to the Lord

Put God in charge of your work, then what you've planned will take place. (Proverbs 16:3 MSG)

Setting goals is a spiritual discipline. Goals stretch you and help you become all God wants you to be. Setting goals will give a destination for your vision. Move forward toward health in all areas of life by creating SMART goals (specific, measurable, attainable, relevant, and time-bound) in response to your results from the Five Essentials survey.

Specific goals are clear. Tell your brain exactly what is expected and why it's important. A specific goal usually answers who, what, when, where, why.

Measurable emphasizes tangible benchmarks. If a goal is not measurable, it is not possible to know whether you are making progress. A measurable goal usually answers how much and by when.

Attainable means the goals need to be realistic, even though dreams can be big. Extreme goals usually invite failure and frustration.

Relevant means you choose goals that matter and answer yes to these questions: Does this seem worthwhile? Is this the right time? Does this match your other efforts/needs? Being relevant also means your goals are relevant to God and bring him glory. Any goal that brings you closer to him and makes you want to serve him and others is a goal that matters.

Time-bound emphasizes attaining the goal within a certain time frame. A deadline helps you focus on completion of the goal on or before the due date.

Once you've determined your SMART goals, share them with a friend. People getting healthy together lose twice as much weight as those who do it alone. That success dramatically increases when you are connected with others, receiving constant encouragement. Consider inviting some friends to do the six-week Daniel Plan study together. Visit *danielplan.com/curriculum/*.

TODAY'S STEPS

1. Set SMART goals and share them with a friend.
2. Complete today's activity in the 40-Day Fitness Challenge, and schedule your exercise for the week.
3. Add real, whole foods to your meals.

Rely on God's Power, Not Willpower

I can do all this through him who gives me strength.
(Philippians 4:13)

When God puts his Spirit inside you, your body becomes a residence for his love. You are not the owner of your body, but a caretaker, or manager, of it. Are you making the most of what you've been given?

The truth is, change and good stewardship are much more sustainable when we focus on what we can have rather than what we can't. Often we subscribe to the misguided notion that change requires deprivation. We easily focus on what we can't have instead of the abundance of things we can enjoy.

If we focus on bringing in the good and enjoying God's abundance, our body, mind, and spirit will become stronger. We will begin to see that things such as walking in the morning or reading our Bible and praying are not things we "have to" do, but opportunities we "get to take hold of" because they rejuvenate and restore us. This is how the perspective shift begins. And it's a good principle to add to your motivation for health.

This perspective can help you cultivate a different relationship with food and fitness. You can start to see eating healthfully as a way to be kind to yourself, to lovingly care for your body. The beauty of adding food that heals, nourishes, and satisfies is that it will almost effortlessly shift your body and mind into a different state — a state where your cravings are gone, where your willpower is not needed because you naturally crave what makes you thrive and feel good. (Visit *goo.gl/ZYjvN4* for a "Good Foods List" to get you started.)

As you exercise today, breathe deeply and thank God for the many blessings he has given you. Ask him to shift your thinking to rely on his power to transform your health and your perspective. Take a couple of stretch breaks throughout your day and repeat this thanksgiving and interaction with God. (See pages 166–69 in *The Daniel Plan* book for ideas.)

TODAY'S STEPS

1. Treat your body like God's temple.
2. Focus on adding good foods to your diet.
3. Thank God for good food and your body.
4. Add stretch breaks to your day.

Design Your Lifestyle

*Prayer: God, where you guide me, I know that you will
provide. What you call me to do, you will equip me to do.
Please remind me of your unending power and resources
to sustain and fulfill me every step of this journey.*

Did you know that people who keep food journals
lose twice as much weight as those who don't?
Journaling is effective not only with food, but with
all five Essentials.

Start using *The Daniel Plan Journal* or a journal of
your own. Write down everything you eat: portion
size, type of food, time, how you feel when eating
it (stress, hunger, boredom, fatigue). Writing down
what you eat does two things: It makes you conscious of what you really are eating, and it helps you
shift and change your habits. What are you eating,
and how does it make you feel?

In terms of fitness, think about one word to
describe your motivation to help you reach your fitness goals. (If you need ideas, see page 155 of *The
Daniel Plan* book.) Jot it down. Then write down any
games, activities, and/or sports you loved to play as a

child. Use these ideas for your daily exercise routine. No matter how big or small, record your exercise accomplishments each day. If you move your body, it's an accomplishment.

One of the best ways to make steady progress is to track your progress. If you ever feel stuck, journal about the negative thoughts that are holding you back. Then head to God's Word to replace them with truth.

Share your journal with your friends, buddy, or small group. You will learn a lot about yourself, and as you do, you will be able to easily make changes that bring healing to your body and mind. What friends can you think of who have a positive influence on your health? Jot their names in your journal, and invite them to join you on this journey. If no one comes to mind, get connected at your local community center or try a new fitness class. Check out the many online resources or social media venues to connect you with people who are committed to living a healthy lifestyle.

Be sure to join our Daniel Plan Facebook page *facebook.com/theDanielPlan*, where we serve up daily inspiration and encouragement.

TODAY'S STEPS

1. Start journaling about food and fitness. Consider journaling about faith and focus as well.
2. Track your progress.

Bring in the Good

Note: The next three days heavily focus on food education and awareness. For maximum long-term benefits, adopt all the principles we outline. If you decide you want to take the fast track, go to Day 9 to start the 10-Day Detox.

We don't count calories on The Daniel Plan, but focus on overall long-term health. When you consume lots of fresh vegetables and low-glycemic fruit, a moderate amount of lean protein, healthy whole grains and healthy fats, your palate will begin to change and you will be able to make better, satisfying food choices without the need to count every calorie. The Daniel Plan is rooted in a simple principle: Take the junk out, and invite the abundance in.

The Daniel Plan is a high-carb diet — but they are unrefined, unprocessed, low-glycemic carbs, otherwise known as vegetables, fruits, whole grains, and beans. (See pages 82–83 in *The Daniel Plan* book for information on the glycemic index.) The Daniel Plan plate is half non-starchy vegetables, one quarter lean protein, and one quarter whole grains or starchy vegetables.

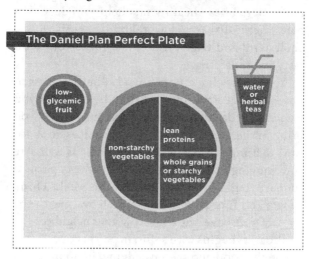

Here are the main concepts to incorporate into your diet now:

Eat from the rainbow of colors in the plant world.

Add whole grains in moderation. Buy them in their original form, such as oats, wheat berries, and even popcorn.

Boost your fiber with whole grains, legumes (beans and peas), and vegetables.

Power up with protein in every meal.

Enjoy healthful fats. Fats from fish, nuts, seeds, avocados, olives and extra virgin olive oil, and coconut butter. These healthy fats help to reduce diabetes, heart disease, cancer, and dementia; lower cholesterol and triglycerides; and make your food tasty and satisfying.

Your daily choices, with God's limitless power, done with a community of friends, can help you launch each day with intention and purpose. As you bring in the good with your food choices, look for ways to bring in the good in your fitness as well. Are you enjoying exercise that you love with people who support you? Try something new this week. Think simple and fun. Maybe a 20-minute walk with the dogs. (Don't have a dog? Borrow your neighbor's!)

Progress begins with a shift in perspective: focusing on the good and acknowledging the abundance.

TODAY'S STEPS

1. Follow The Daniel Plan plate at every meal.
2. Add fiber, color, whole grains, protein, and good fats to your food choices.
3. Choose an exercise you enjoy.

Create Your Daniel Plan Kitchen

Prayer: Father, help me to accept that many man-made foods are addictive and cause harm to my body. Transform my mind to care for my body and embrace the truth that many foods are good for my body, mind, and spirit. Lord, through your power I know I can change and embrace the abundance you have provided.

Clean out your kitchen. Out with the old, and in with the new! The first step in creating a Daniel Plan pantry, fridge, and freezer is to clean out the stuff that is not serving you well. This means reading labels, checking expiration dates, and tossing the bad stuff, then refilling with healthy new items — which you have already been adding to your diet. Simply getting rid of harmful foods from your eating life will make a tremendous difference in your health and eating habits. Do this with your dry pantry, where you store canned goods, whole grains, and nonperishables. Then go through your refrigerator and freezer too.

To start, read labels for unhealthy ingredients. Aim for labels with five ingredients or less, or at least ingredients that you recognize as real food. (Go to Day 17 for more on reading labels.)

- Remove anything that says HFCS (High Fructose Corn Syrup), MSG (Monosodium Glutamate), trans fats (partially hydrogenated and hydrogenated fats).
- Banish sugary breakfast cereals, unhealthy cookies and crackers, fried chips, and junk food.
- Exile high-sugar or high-sodium condiments.
- Evict unhealthy oils, such as standard mass-market "vegetable" oil and shortening.
- Say goodbye to the "white menaces": white sugar, white flour, white rice, and white pasta. These white foods act like sugar in the body. Bottom line: Sugar is an occasional treat. When you have sugar, stick with traditional natural forms: raw sugar, raw honey, natural fruit sugars, or pure maple syrup.
- Discard liquid calories: regular and diet sodas, sports drinks and other sweetened beverages, juice.
- Remove foods with the following additives: artificial sweeteners (except stevia), sodium and calcium caseinate, soy protein isolate,

phosphoric acid, sulfites, nitrates/nitrites, artificial colors, flavors and dyes, and carrageenan.

Now breathe a big sigh of relief. You just removed dozens of harmful foods from your kitchen. Your body and mind will thank you. Don't forget to record this big move in your journal and share it with your friends.

TODAY'S STEP

Clean out your pantry, refrigerator, and freezer.

Eat Foods That Love You Back

But I am like an olive tree flourishing in the house of God; I trust in God's unfailing love for ever and ever. (Psalm 52:8)

Congratulations, you took a huge step yesterday! Today you will restock your kitchen with delicious, good-for-you foods.

Start a shopping list of food staples that you should always have on hand. Pick and choose items based on your taste preferences, but don't be afraid to try new foods. Some everyday ingredients will save you in a pinch and ensure that you are prepared to put together a quick, healthy meal in a matter of minutes:

- Chopped vegetables
- Fresh greens (make your own custom mix for salads or to complement your morning smoothie)
- Berries (add to smoothies, oatmeal, or salads)

- Avocados (add to smoothies, grains, or salads)
- Alternative milks (as a base for smoothies, coffee, or lattes)

Now make a list of staples to add to your pantry. With a well-stocked pantry, you will never be at a loss for something healthy to eat. (See pages 15–16 and 28 in *The Daniel Plan Cookbook* for nonstarchy vegetable ideas, low-sugar fruits, and easy replacements and alternatives.) Here are a few basics:

FOR SNACKS AND MEALS
- Whole grain or brown rice crackers
- Baked corn, baked vegetable, or brown rice chips
- Bean-based and vegetable puree soups, and soups made with alternative healthy milks
- Nuts, nut butters, dark chocolate
- Guacamole, hummus, tzatziki, salsa
- Herbal teas, water with citrus wedges

FOR COOKING
- Unrefined, cold-pressed, and expeller-pressed oils
- Whole grain wheat flour, organic sprouted almond flour, gluten-free flour, or organic cornmeal

- Old-fashioned oats, steel cut oats, buckwheat, or kasha
- Whole wheat, brown rice pasta, or quinoa pasta
- Brown or black rice, quinoa, barley

These are foods that love you back. (Find more in the "Top 10 Choices in Each Food Group" on page 80 of *The Daniel Plan* book.) And The Daniel Plan is built on love as the motivation: Experiencing God's unconditional love for you, learning to love him back, learning to love foods and exercise that love you back, and learning to give and receive love from others. It is love — not fear, not guilt, and not peer pressure — that causes us to keep going when we feel like giving up.

TODAY'S STEPS

1. Stock your pantry with foods that love you back.
2. Focus on love as your motivation for health.

Jumpstart Your Success

So whether you eat or drink or whatever you do, do it all for the glory of God. (1 Corinthians 10:31)

If you really want to take it up a notch and get fast results (health or weight), we highly encourage that you start with a 10-day (which you can extend to 40 days) Daniel Plan Detox to jumpstart the healing process, reboot your system, and discover the power of reclaiming your body and mind. With the detox you let go of the things that can harm you and add in the things that can heal you (which you've already been putting into action over the past few days). There may be foods in your diet that are working against your health, creating inflammation, and preventing you from releasing weight and/or overcoming chronic health issues. Using the power of healing foods, your body and mind will quickly transform, and you will realize just how well you can feel and how quickly it can happen.

Why do The Daniel Plan Detox? Many of us

usually feel less than fully healthy. We either have nagging complaints such as fatigue and brain fog or more serious conditions. By giving your body a chance to reset for a short period of time, you will learn firsthand the power of food to heal and the abundance, energy, and vibrancy that can come from a healing way of eating. Here are some of the benefits you may experience in just a few weeks:

- Weight loss of 5 – 10 pounds or more
- Better digestion and elimination
- Fewer symptoms of chronic illness
- Improved concentration, mental focus, and clarity
- Improved mood and increased sense of internal balance
- Increased energy and sense of well-being
- Less congestion and fewer allergic symptoms
- Less fluid retention
- Less joint pain
- Increased sense of peace and relaxation
- Enhanced sleep
- Improved skin

If you aren't ready for the detox, that's okay. We offer a core meal plan if you decide you want to take it slower. The core plan is based on the DP plate and will work long-term for whole health through real food. (See chapter 10 of *The Daniel Plan* book for both meal plans.)

No matter which plan you choose, trust God's power to strengthen you, and ask for support from the friends or family who are with you on this journey.

TODAY'S STEPS

1. Start The Daniel Plan 10-Day or 40-Day Detox or the core meal plan.
2. Enlist support from friends.

Shop Smart

If you think shopping is a chore, hopefully Daniel Plan shopping will change your mind. Consider it as an errand that boosts your health by stocking up on foods that heal. It can also be fun. Whether at a farmer's market; grocery, specialty, or health store; CSA (community-supported agriculture); food co-ops; or online — buying healthy ingredients that taste good can motivate you to get into the kitchen and cook.

Before you go shopping, you can shift your mindset into a place of truth. Grab your journal and jot down any triggers, foods that have the potential to trip you up, and what thoughts surround those foods. Then make sure they don't wind up on your list or in your cart.

Grab a shopping list for either the core or detox meal plans from chapter 10 of *The Daniel Plan* book. Or simply follow these tips:

1. Shop the perimeter. The perimeter of the market is where the produce, eggs, meat, and seafood departments are located.

2. Buy in bulk to save money.
3. Brave the inside aisles. Although there are many aisles that you now can totally skip, and that will save you time (and money!), the inside aisles are where you will find packaged whole grains, canned beans, frozen berries and vegetables, healthy oils, vinegars, dried herbs and spices, packaged nuts, broths, and condiments.
4. Keep it cool. When you buy fresh seafood, ask for ice to keep it cold until you get home. And use insulated shopping bags to help keep cold things cold.
5. Stock up, wisely. Be smart about how much you can store and how much you will practically use. This includes frozen items such as berries for smoothies and fresh, ground meat and poultry that will keep when wrapped well (or vacuum-sealed) in the freezer. Nuts, which can be expensive, store in the freezer for up to six months when wrapped well or vacuum-sealed.

Not only is food medicine, but so is community. Community is the cure to much of what ails us. We get better together.

There's a wonderful word in the original language

of the New Testament that is used to describe the community of the early church: *koinonia*. It is most often translated "fellowship," a word we sometimes tend to use as a synonym for socializing, perhaps with our church friends. But *koinonia* means far more than mere socializing or even gathering in a small group. It means love, intimacy, and joyful participation, deep communion with one another — putting others' needs before your own. It's a radical level of friendship and community.

TODAY'S STEPS

1. Shop differently, using the tips to find foods that serve as medicine.
2. Challenge yourself to create *koinonia* in your friendships.
3. Turn the page to pause, celebrate, and recalibrate.

Pause, Celebrate, and Recalibrate

Congratulations! You have made incredible progress in setting the stage for your success. You are eating foods that heal, moving your body, and making healthier choices.

- Celebrate where you are today. Then take a few minutes to revisit your goals to see what you've accomplished in these first 10 days!
- Reflect on any setbacks or challenges you have experienced and explore what happened and how you can prepare to avoid them in the next 10 days. Remind yourself of your motivation, the why behind your desire to get healthy.
- Check in with your buddy to share your insight and offer support in their journey as well.

Prayer: God, thank you for helping me day by day as I seek to create a healthy lifestyle. I know that each step I take in the right direction is progress, and ultimately I honor you when I take care of myself. Through your power I can accomplish anything. Develop in me the self-control I need to stay focused and make wise choices.

Looking ahead: Now that you have set the stage for a healthy lifestyle, the next 10 days will help you set a pace for your journey. A doable, consistent pace is important because it provides a foundation for long-term health. Bit by bit you will make progress as you discover movement you enjoy, renew your mind with truth and new perspectives, plan for long-term success, and enlist friends. Even if you face setbacks, you will discover that they are not failures, but simply opportunities to learn and apply in the days to come.

Discover Movement You Enjoy

For in him we live and move and have our being.
(Acts 17:28)

When we were young, moving our bodies was a natural part of our day. We looked forward to recess. We longed for it. We dreamt about it. Back then we called it "play," and we loved every minute of it. Today, for many, we call it "exercise" and count every minute of it, longing for it to be over. We frequently find it painful, boring, or dull, and we feel guilty about not doing it.

Kay Warren said, "You were meant for something more. You were meant to experience a life of joy." Our days are spent with long spans of minimal movement, which impacts not only our joy, but also our bodies. Yet many of us won't switch to an active lifestyle just because it's good for us.

So what will change us? Discovering movement we enjoy. "Play."

Take a moment to think about your main motivation to propel you toward a lifetime of health. To help you through this process, we want you to think about your reason a little bit differently.

In the book *One Word That Will Change Your Life*, the authors (Dan Britton, Jimmy Page, and Jon Gordon) present the idea of focusing on one word every year to help transform your life. We can apply this wisdom to finding one word for the changes you want to make on The Daniel Plan. For example, if your dream is to run the Boston Marathon, your one-word reason may be *challenge* or *accomplishment*. Maybe your dream is to start a hiking club and tour different parts of the world, so your word might be *enjoyment* or *fellowship*.

What one word comes to mind for why you want to achieve your particular fitness dream?

Take the one word motivation and apply it to your eating choices and your daily quiet time with God. Let this word guide you as you sit down to a meal. Chew your food slowly, and think of how it is building your health. Enjoy the benefits.

Doing what you enjoy, with the help of God and others, you will gain the motivation, encouragement, direction, and strength to help you become Daniel Strong. And let us know how you're doing. Join us on social media: @TheDanielPlan Facebook, Twitter, Instagram, or Pinterest.

TODAY'S STEPS

1. Incorporate movement you enjoy into the 40-Day Fitness Challenge.
2. Find one word to motivate your health and your fitness plan.
3. Join The Daniel Plan on social media.

Be Transformed by the Renewing of Your Mind

Do not conform to the pattern of this world, but be transformed by the renewing of your mind.
(Romans 12:2)

Commit this verse to memory. It will be a focal point and anchor in your journey.

With one decision — an action made by your brain — you began a journey to wellness that offers you increased energy, lower stress, and better sleep (among the many other benefits you have already read about). We want that one decision to last for a lifetime, which requires a renewed mind and sustained focus. In a world where so many distractions compete for your attention, it is more important than ever to stop the busyness in your head and focus on God's plan and priorities for your life.

Unfortunately, it is the loss of focus that causes many people to cycle through hopeful starts and many failed stops as other things vie for their attention.

Identify and challenge your thought patterns through journaling. Tracking your success as well as making note of any challenges or modifications allows you to identify any ongoing negative thoughts, behaviors, or patterns that may undermine your efforts toward better health.

Whether you use *The Daniel Plan Journal*, an e-journal, or a notebook, we encourage you to record your journey. Looking back through your daily entries can be motivating as you reflect on all the headway you've made. Reflecting on your journey also helps you figure out your next small step. As Pastor Rick Warren often says, you cannot manage what you do not measure. Journaling your progress is practical, and as you make progress, you will be motivated to continue.

Another essential that keeps you on track and helps you focus is your friends. Did you know that your social circles influence your health even more than your DNA? We are more likely to be overweight if our friends are, even if our parents are not. At the same time, we are more likely to exercise and eat healthy food, to not smoke or overeat, if our friends also practice healthy habits. If they are sick, we are more likely to be sick. If our friends have healthy habits, then we probably will also.

So let Romans 12:2, a journal, and your friends

boost your confidence and motivation as you move forward one step at a time.

TODAY'S STEPS

1. Meditate on Romans 12:2. Commit this verse to memory.
2. Identify and challenge your thought patterns through journaling.
3. Thank God for your progress.

Plan for Success

Improving our health is possible, but doing so requires intention and effort in our daily choices. When we choose to spend time with God, to exercise, to eat healthy food, and to focus our thoughts, we take steps toward our goals in every area of life.

One of the biggest keys to your success is planning. By intentionally planning for the week, you create space in your busy week and prioritize your efforts before they happen. You can plan your quiet time, your food choices, your fitness, and your connections with friends. Planning is a powerful way to set you up for healthy choices time and time again.

For example, every Sunday evening exercise physiologist Sean Foy sits down with his phone calendar and schedules his fitness for the week. Many of his clients follow the same ritual. These are nonnegotiable appointments that Foy makes with either his fitness buddies or himself.

A food plan will help you get into the habit of putting together balanced, wholesome nourishment that's easy for your everyday routine. Simple tips include cutting up veggies, making hummus and healthy dips, portioning out nuts for snacks, boiling eggs, pre-cooking a grain, or preparing chicken or wild tuna/salmon that you can toss onto a salad.

Planning will also help you avoid a food emergency. What is a food emergency? When your blood sugar starts to drop, you are hard-wired to eat anything (and everything) in sight. A few tips that will keep you from facing a food emergency include starting your day with a healthy balanced breakfast, eating every three to four hours, hydrating your body throughout the day, and stocking an emergency food pack.

We recommend that everyone create an emergency food pack; it will be your food safety net. Find your favorite things to include; the choices are plentiful. Stock these packs in your home, your travel bag or purse, your car, and your workplace with key rations for any food emergency. (Check out page 53 in *The Daniel Plan Cookbook* for more time-saving tips and ideas on how to prepare and plan for your week.)

TODAY'S STEPS

1. Take time today to plan your meals and snacks for the week.
2. Create an emergency food pack.

3. Make appointments for your fitness routine based on the 40-Day Fitness Challenge. How has the fitness plan changed how you feel physically? Emotionally? Journal your thoughts.

Friends are the Secret Sauce

As iron sharpens iron, so a friend sharpens a friend.
(Proverbs 27:17 NLT)

When you have God and a group helping you, you now have far more than willpower helping you to make positive changes, and you are far more likely to stay consistent. Involving your friends is not just a feel-good aspect of The Daniel Plan. Research backs up the concept, showing how crucial we are for each other's healing and success. Much of what currently ails us (and people all over the globe) is preventable, treatable, and very often curable. Even better: the cure is right next to us.

You already have community in some way. You may have a prayer circle that supports your spiritual walk. You may meet with a dinner club in which everyone finds joy in cooking. You may be part of a moms or dads group where you all talk about the daily challenges of raising your kids. You have friends who support you.

God made you to thrive when you're connected with others. Being engaged in community will improve your health — and not just physically. Friends can improve your emotional and spiritual health.

The opposite is also true: Isolation injures us. Our lack of community can keep us from being the healthiest we can be. In other words, the Friends Essential is the "secret sauce" for all the other Essentials.

One of the reasons The Daniel Plan has already helped thousands of people create a healthier lifestyle is the fact that it is done in community. When we introduced The Daniel Plan, more than 15,000 people joined small groups in person or online, eager to find friends who could help them. Each group had its own focus and flavor.

One group of women not only met to study and pray together, but once a week would also shop together for healthy food. They would go back to one woman's house and cook in bulk. They would divide up the food and each take home a few premade meals.

Touch base with your friend(s) who are also on the journey toward better health. Ask if you can start meeting as a group for regular exercise, meals, or study. Consider starting *The Daniel Plan DVD and Study Guide* together.

TODAY'S STEPS

1. Touch base with your friends about sharing a health-oriented activity together or supporting one another through prayer.
2. Consider starting a Daniel Plan group.
3. Pray about sharing your story with us about becoming healthier. You can email us at *info@danielplan.com*.

Replace Negative Thoughts

The Daniel Plan focuses on abundance, not deprivation. That requires learning some new thinking skills, such as replacing negative thoughts with truth rather than resisting them. The more you fight a feeling, the more it controls you. The secret of victory over any temptation is simply to change the channel of your mind. Refocus your attention on something else, and the temptation immediately loses its power.

Every time you have a thought, your brain releases chemicals. Negative, angry, and hopeless thoughts produce negative chemicals that make your body and mind feel bad; by contrast, positive, happy, and hopeful thoughts produce a completely different set of chemicals that help you feel relaxed, happy, and in control of your impulses.

Whenever you feel sad, mad, nervous, or out of control, identify which of the types of the negative thoughts you are engaging in. Challenge the negative thoughts by finding and stating the truth. This takes away their power and gives you control over your thoughts, moods, and behaviors.

When Solange Montoya started The Daniel Plan with two friends, she was hoping to change more than her weight and how her clothes fit. She knew there was more to lifelong health. And there was!

"So many insecurities and all this negative self-talk come when you don't feel like you can do this physically," she says. "But there was such a change when I had that energy and [started thinking positively instead of negatively]. I just feel like, *Wow, God, there's nothing now that I don't want to do for you.* The excuses just kind of started to melt away, more so than the weight."

The good news is that a life of abundance and vitality is right around the corner. With each healthy choice, you step closer to your goals. The more you focus on the abundance of choices, the more it boosts your motivation and commitment.

> **Prayer:** *Lord, help me believe that you have good plans for me, plans of abundance and hope. When I get stuck in negative thinking and lies, direct me to your truth to renew my mind and my thoughts. Teach me to remember your promise in Jeremiah 29:11, embracing the truth that you have prosperous plans for my future.*

TODAY'S STEP

Journal about any negative thoughts that trouble
you. Next to each one replace it with truth. (See
page 204 in *The Daniel Plan* book for examples.)

No Such Thing As Failure

Lord, when doubts fill my mind, when my heart is in turmoil, quiet me and give me renewed hope and cheer. (Psalm 94:19 TLB)

Your attitude toward failure will determine your ultimate success. Focus and a healthy mind can help you reframe setbacks as opportunities to learn and recalibrate.

Expect both ups and downs on your journey toward better health. There will be highlights and setbacks. Failure does not have to defeat or derail you. It can actually increase your chances of ultimate success. The Daniel Plan encourages you to turn bad days into good information and to study your failures. Learn from your mistakes.

Regardless of your circumstances and how you feel, focus on who God is — his unchanging nature. Remind yourself of what you know to be eternally true about God: *He is good, he loves me, he is for me.*

He knows my struggles and my circumstances, and I know he has a good plan for my life.

Setbacks help you identify your most vulnerable moments. We do not want you to be a victim of your failures, but rather to study them to understand what contributed to the outcome. Be curious. We like saying, "Turn bad days into good data."

Follow a few simple rules for vulnerable times:

- Manage your stress.
- Avoid your triggers.
- Eat healthy foods first.
- When tempted, take a walk, repeat a poem or Scripture verse, drink a glass of water.
- Be aware of impulses and then focus on something else until the impulse goes away.
- Get 7 to 8 hours of sleep.
- Get moving.

Follow the 90/10 rule. Give yourself a break. Make great food choices 90 percent of the time, and allow yourself margin to enjoy some of your favorite foods on occasion. This way you won't feel deprived, and you will avoid binging on something you'll regret later.

As you shift your perspective on failure, liberate your friends by showing them grace. Encourage and support others when they make mistakes or hit a rut on their journey. When people know they are loved, you can become a safe place where your friends feel free to share their challenges and find the confidence to turn their setbacks around.

TODAY'S STEPS

1. Think about a setback that happened recently, that you initially considered a failure. Turn it around. How can you use this for tomorrow? (For an example, see page 202 in *The Daniel Plan* book.)
2. Call or write a friend and ask how you can support them when they face setbacks.

Focus on What's True

All Scripture is inspired by God and is useful to teach us what is true and to make us realize what is wrong in our lives. It corrects us when we are wrong and teaches us to do what is right. (2 Timothy 3:16 NLT)

Is it true?" Carry these words with you everywhere you go. They can interrupt your thoughts and short-circuit an episode of bingeing, depression, or even panic. One of our participants weighed 425 pounds when he first joined The Daniel Plan. When one of the doctors asked him about his weight, his automatic response was, "I have no control."

"Is it true?" the doctor asked. "You really have NO control over your eating?"

The man paused then said, "No. That really isn't true; I do have some control."

When you stop believing lies and replace them with accurate thinking and God's truth and promises, your response to life events will shift, and you will feel less stressed and more hopeful. (For examples of filling your mind with truth, see pages 204–7 of *The Daniel Plan* book.)

On a practical level, use truth to make discerning choices about your food. Read labels, not just the advertising on the front. Watch out for health claims. Anything with a health claim is almost guaranteed to be bad for you — diet this or low-fat that or trans fat — free or low calorie or cholesterol lowering.

The nutrition label is your new best friend. If you follow these simple rules, you will stay out of trouble:

- If there are any words on the label that you don't recognize or can't pronounce, are in Latin, or sound like some science project, then put the product back on the shelf.
- Think five or less ingredients. Some newer healthier products contain more, but they are all real food.
- Be alert to pseudonyms for sugar. (See page 108 in *The Daniel Plan* book for a list of names for sugar.)
- What comes first? Ingredients are listed in order of quantity. If you see sugar or salt as the first or second ingredient, find another option.

The more you find and state the truth, the more knowledge and control you will have over your thoughts and behaviors in any area of your life.

TODAY'S STEPS

1. Practice asking yourself, "Is it true?"
2. Start reading nutrition labels on every food item before purchase.

Healthy Brain, Healthy Body

But test everything that is said. Hold on to what is good. (1 Thessalonians 5:21 NLT)

Your brain is the most amazing organ. Even though it is only 2 percent of your body's weight, it uses 20 to 30 percent of the calories you consume and 20 percent of the oxygen and blood flow in your body. It is the most expensive real estate in your body, requiring the most resources.

Practice using your brain. Self-control is like a muscle. The more you use it, the stronger it gets. Just as good parents help children develop self-control by saying no, strengthen the self-control part of your own brain by saying no to the things that are not good for you. Over time your brain will make better choices more automatically. (For more brain-boosting tips, see pages 222–23 in *The Daniel Plan* book.)

As you boost the health of your brain, take new steps to boost the health of your body. Incorporate some new food and fitness concepts into your Daniel Plan lifestyle.

First, beware of health food impostors: sweetened yogurt, processed/genetically modified soy products, meat alternatives, protein bars, and fruit juice. (See page 142 of *The Daniel Plan* book for more information.)

Second, if your budget allows, eat organic to avoid pesticides, hormones, and antibiotics in food. Use the Clean Fifteen and Dirty Dozen list from the Environmental Working Group (*ewg.org*) to choose the least contaminated conventionally grown fruits and vegetables and avoid the most contaminated versions. Look for the terms grass fed, pasture raised, free-range or organic, or made without hormones and antibiotics. If more people choose organics, the prices will come down.

Third, combat sitting disease. Did you know the average person sits 7.7-15 hours a day? Just moving more often during your day can make a big difference to your health! Go to *goo.gl/DFLRW5* for a 2-minute micro break you can use during your busy day.

Effective decisions involve forethought in relation to your goals, which helps you live life to the fullest today, while supporting plans for your future. Boosting your brain power and optimizing your health will help you maximize your decision-making ability.

TODAY'S STEPS

1. With God's help, practice self-control in your eating habits and thought patterns.
2. Avoid health food impostors and incorporate organic foods.
3. Take 2-minute micro breaks to move your body throughout the day.

Small Steps = Big Results

Prayer: Lord, please help me to be energetic in my salvation and to find that energy from you (Philippians 2:12 – 13). As I face each day, remind me that my strength comes from you and that any small step toward better health is a step that will honor you.

The key to a faith-filled life is not in trying harder. It's not in psyching yourself up, but in relaxing in God's grace.

What's most important is that you are taking small steps in the right direction. Many began The Daniel Plan by simply trying a new health habit, just one small thing. They decided to start the day with breakfast, or add more veggies to their meals, or take a brisk walk each day, or invite a friend to work out. Small steps, yes. But they began to see surprising life change. Simple changes started to add up. Small steps took them closer to realizing their big dreams.

A gradual approach is the surest way to success. Trying to change everything at once almost inevitably invites disappointment. Don't try to change dozens of unhealthy habits at once. Start with a few vital behaviors — the ones that will have the biggest immediate impact — and go from there. Here are a few small steps to try if you haven't incorporated them yet:

- Set a goal in faith to take time in God's Word and be refreshed by his promises.
- Start walking with friends.
- Eat breakfast every day. (See chapter 10 of *The Daniel Plan* book or *The Daniel Plan Cookbook* for recipe ideas.)
- Eat some protein with every meal.
- Drink water. Half your body weight in ounces.
- Pray before your meals.
- Thank God for your body while you are stretching or taking a micro break.
- Take 2-minute micro breaks to move your body throughout the day.
- Try a new aerobic activity.

A key to The Daniel Plan is remembering that small steps lead to big results. This week, tell a friend or your Daniel Plan group about one small-step or positive outcome you have experienced.

TODAY'S STEPS

1. Remind yourself that small steps = big results.
2. Add one small step to your new healthy lifestyle this week.

Progress, Not Perfection

Prayer: Lord, will you remind me that perfection is never the goal but a heart toward you and your ways? Help me to feel secure, knowing that getting healthy is a matter of making progress, one healthy choice at a time. I trust that your strength will give me confident hope, patience in hard times, and the faithfulness to keep praying. (Romans 12:12)

When your progress wavers, pay attention. What causes setbacks with your food or fitness? Is it when you get too busy? Is it when you don't get enough sleep? Notice patterns, cycles, and reactions — not to make yourself feel guilty, but so you have valuable information from which to make healthier decisions in the future.

We all make mistakes. When we track our victories as well as setbacks, we see that God's grace is sufficient, and his love is bigger than any of our weaknesses. If you have a bad day with any of the Essentials, don't be upset; instead, view that as a great opportunity to learn to use as insight for tomorrow.

One of the best ways to make steady progress is to track your progress. (For ideas, go to page 176 in *The Daniel Plan* book.) To help you make consistent daily, weekly, and monthly progress, monitoring and/or tracking your efforts is important. In fact, in multiple studies, individuals who monitored their exercise habits significantly improved their behavior and likelihood of accomplishing their goals.

When it comes to food, a choice as simple as smart snacking can show you how daily progress builds momentum and leads to long-term success. Smart snacking means choosing something with protein and avoiding sugar. Here are some great grab-and-go ideas:

- Stock your fridge with healthy dips (hummus, guacamole), low-sugar fruits, Greek yogurt, and hard-boiled eggs.
- Carry a small cooler and ice packs in your car for food items that need to stay cold.
- Toss together a bean salad with olive oil, herbs, salt, pepper, and spices such as cumin, onion, or shallot.
- Stock mini-packets of nut butters.
- Stock healthy jerky (salmon, turkey, grass-fed beef, bison, organic, without added nitrates or MSG).

- Make organic air-popped popcorn.
- Drink plenty of water. Sometimes you are dehydrated, not hungry.

As you focus on progress, not perfection, you will be equipped to run the race God has set for you. Trust him, and trust the friends who are with you on this journey. Be brave enough to be authentic — to reveal your issues and graciously accept the weaknesses of others. Foster a community where every friend is not afraid to ask for help — starting with yourself.

TODAY'S STEPS

1. Journal about your progress (see the next page, "Pause, Celebrate, and Recalibrate").
2. Make smart snacks to have on hand.

Pause, Celebrate, and Recalibrate

Congratulations! You are halfway through your 40-day start toward a healthier life.

Celebrate how much you have learned over the past 20 days. Praise God for his faithfulness in the process. Revisit Day 12 and meditate on Romans 12:2. Express your gratitude for how each healthy step you take brings you closer to your goals.

- Reflect on any setbacks or challenges you have experienced, and explore what happened and how you can prepare to avoid them in the next 10 days. Reframe them as learning versus failure. A setback is just an opportunity for a comeback.
- Check in with your buddy. Together, revisit your goals and your motivation and talk about your progress and learning opportunities. Offer encouragement and support in your buddy's journey as well. Remember, we get better together.

Looking ahead: Now that you have set your pace, you are ready to enter the second half of this 40-day experience as you learn to make room for grace. Let go of any tendencies to seek perfection, for that is not God's will for you. God's greatest desire is for you to live in the peace that grace brings to your body, mind, and spirit. As you maximize your energy, turn to God for strength, implement the power of gratitude, and enjoy the benefits this new lifestyle brings, be mindful of what a little of gentleness can do.

Grace and Pace

But [God] said to me, "My grace is sufficient for you, for my power is made perfect in weakness." Therefore I will boast all the more gladly about my weaknesses, so that Christ's power may rest on me. (2 Corinthians 12:9)

If you were to ask ten people if they believe exercise is good for their health and well-being, how many of them do you think would raise their hands? If you guessed nine out of ten, you would match what we all intuitively know to be true. Exercise is good for us. But what do you think is the number one exercise that will help you feel younger, ramp up a sluggish metabolism, reduce and manage your weight, boost your energy, increase cardiovascular endurance, improve muscular tone and strength, enhance sleep, reduce stress, and bring joy and youthfulness back to your life?

The number one exercise to help you attain all of these benefits ... is the one you will do! It's true. Despite all the research surrounding the benefits of regular exercise, the only one that will make a difference is the program you will do consistently.

But we have a problem. Only about half of us exercise three or more days a week. The amazing health and life-changing benefits of exercise we all know about don't motivate the majority of us to get off the sofa or easy chair and move.

Let's get to the bottom of this. What if you wanted to exercise? What if you were inspired and truly motivated to lace up your gym shoes and go for a walk, a run, or a hike? What if you moved from thinking, *I know I should exercise* to *I can't wait to exercise* and, by integrating motion with devotion, you could grow closer and stronger in your relationship with God? What if you discovered the moves that made you feel younger and recapture the joy and fun of your youth?

Throughout your week, thank God for the many blessings he has given you. Take a couple of stretch breaks throughout the day to remember that this journey is about grace and pace. It's not a sprint, nor a final destination. Stay the course and continue completing your daily Daniel Strong challenges in the book. When you allow God to change your mind from a "have to" mentality to a "get to," it allows room for grace and pace for yourself and for others. Encourage and affirm the friends who are with you on this journey toward health. (For a list of ways to support each other, see page 241 in *The Daniel Plan* book.)

Point out the progress they've made. Even a short text can make the world of difference as they make their way through the day.

TODAY'S STEPS

1. Meditate on 2 Corinthians 12:9.
2. Take several stretch breaks throughout the day.
3. Encourage and affirm your friends.

Follow the 90/10 Rule

It's worth saying again: Don't beat yourself up about setbacks. You may default to negative thinking and find yourself thinking you have failed. That's the human condition. Recognize it for what it is, and make the decision to focus on all the progress you have made.

To avoid setbacks and help you stay on track, adopt the *90/10 rule.* This guideline simply means that 90 percent of the time you are making healthy choices. Then give yourself a 10 percent margin to make choices just for fun. Don't stress about it. Just enjoy it.

To stay focused on eating well and still enjoying a vibrant social life, here are some basic strategies:

- Never go to a party hungry. If you have a snack before, you won't be tempted to eat every greasy, fried, or sugary food.
- Eat before you travel. Never go to an airport, a ballgame, or a public event hungry.
- Bring your food. If you are going to a picnic, bring healthy options to avoid being tempted with unhealthy choices.

- Start a trend with your friends. See who can find the best real food in your town. You can read menus online and make sure there are healthy choices.
- Stock up on the road. If you are traveling, stock up on healthy snacks or restock your emergency food pack.
- Start a supper club with your friends or church group. Rotate hosting the meal once a month between friends. Do a potluck or cook recipes from *The Daniel Plan*, *danielplan.com/food*, or *The Daniel Plan Cookbook*.
- Say no to food pushers. These are people who say, "Come on, just have one bite" or "One can of soda can't hurt you." They might feel bad about themselves and want you to join. Don't submit to the momentary pressure; just say, "No thanks!"

Always remember: It's about progress, not perfection. Leave room to be human.

> **Prayer:** *God, I am certain that you began a good work in me and that you will continue your work until it is finished (Philippians 1:6). Thank you for faithfully working in my heart, mind, and body.*

TODAY'S STEPS

1. Follow the 90/10 rule.
2. Try a few of the basic strategies for eating well.

Enjoy Refreshment

"Come to me, all you who are weary and burdened, and I will give you rest." (Matthew 11:28)

When we're overtired, we often try to boost our energy with caffeine, sugar, or carbs, which ultimately leaves us more tired than before. Jesus relaxed, and he offered his followers both physical and spiritual rest. If he didn't sacrifice rest but offered it as a gift, shouldn't we accept that gift? Turn to him for rest.

Relax. The simplest and fastest way to relax and reduce cortisol is to take five breaths. Count to five on the in breath, and count to five on the out breath. Do it five times. Another simple way to relax is to use calming scents. The scent of lavender (or try geranium, rose, cardamom, sandalwood, and chamomile) has been used since ancient times for its calming, stress-relieving properties. This popular aroma reduces cortisol levels and promotes relaxation and stress reduction.

Refresh. Water is life. Because our bodies are 55 to 75 percent water, staying hydrated is paramount to being healthy. Water helps regulate our blood pressure and body temperature, helps improve circulation, and impacts heart rate. Water raises our metabolism, helps us to feel full, removes wastes, lubricates joints, and boosts energy. Water helps prevent muscle cramping, flushes out impurities, and gives our skin a glow. When we don't get enough water, we may feel hungry, tired, and mentally foggy or get a headache.

If you like the fizz of soda, try sparkling water or mineral water. For flavor, add a squeeze of lemon, lime, or orange. Add a little natural juice such as pomegranate or watermelon juice (puree watermelon chunks in the blender and strain) mixed with lime. Add fresh mint leaves or a cucumber slice for a refreshing option.

Rest. Make sure you get enough sleep. Sleep at least 7 to 8 hours a night. Even losing one or two hours of sleep a night can cause you to crave more carbs, and you will end up eating more during the day. Sleep is God's gift; to accept that gift is an act of trust. Restful sleep gives us the energy to exercise. It sharpens our focus and helps us to make good choices about food.

TODAY'S STEPS

1. Spend a few extra minutes in God's Word today.
2. Do something simple to relax.
3. Drink plenty of water.
4. Plan to go to bed early enough to get 7–8 hours sleep.

Not All Calories Are Equal

According to the laws of physics, a calorie is a calorie — the amount of energy required to raise the temperature of one liter of water by one degree centigrade. But all bets are off when you put biology in the mix. There are different kinds of calories: healing calories and disease-causing calories.

Let's compare a 20-ounce soda with 240 calories to the equivalent number of calories from broccoli (which is about 7.5 cups). The soda has no nutritional value, but has 15 teaspoons of sugar (high fructose corn syrup), caffeine, and phosphoric acid. The broccoli (if you could actually eat the 7.5 cups!) has the same number of calories, but about 1/2 teaspoon natural sugar and 35 grams fiber and is rich in vitamins and minerals. In fact, when it enters your body, the broccoli has the exact opposite effect of the soda. Same calories — very different result.

Clearly, all calories are not the same. So we want to help you focus on becoming a "qualitarian."

The Glycemic Index (GI) identifies how carbohydrates affect your blood sugar levels. Carbs with a low GI (55 or less) don't make your blood sugar levels rise too high, but provide sustained energy. Low-glycemic foods include zucchini, spinach, artichokes, berries, peaches, apples, and many more. (Check out the "Top 10 Tips for Low-Glycemic Eating" on pages 82–83 in *The Daniel Plan* book.)

Phytonutrients. An entire class of compounds (phytonutrients) is in our plant foods that reduce inflammation; rid our bodies of toxins; improve the way our bodies metabolize food and boost calorie burning; optimize immune function; and prevent cancer, heart disease, diabetes, and dementia. Think "binge" on vegetables.

Antioxidants. Foods rich in antioxidants prevent aging and promote overall health. They are found in black rice, beets, and pomegranates; orange and yellow vegetables; dark green, leafy vegetables; and fruits such as purple grapes, blueberries, cranberries, and cherries.

Protein. The secret to fewer cravings is getting high quality protein in every meal. A serving size is 4 to 6 ounces or about the size of your palm. (Check out pages 91–95 in *The Daniel Plan* book to learn about the best sources of protein.)

Many foods high in phytonutrients are also

considered superfoods. These are foods richest in high-quality protein, good fats, vitamins, and minerals. These are among the most health-promoting of all the foods you can eat.

TODAY'S STEPS

1. Eat at least five to nine servings a day from the rainbow of non-starchy vegetables.
2. Try a superfood.
3. Buy quality protein and eat smaller portions.

U-Turns Allowed

So now there is no condemnation for those who belong to Christ Jesus. (Romans 8:1 NLT)

On The Daniel Plan you cannot fail — because you start it as a 40-day journey and then get to see changes gradually unfold over your lifetime. You get better ... your momentum builds momentum. You may have a slipup, but you continue moving forward. Setbacks and comebacks are part of the journey, and graciousness is woven through both.

There is no condemnation for those who belong to Christ Jesus. That means God will never condemn you. He wants you to succeed! He's walking with you every step of the way and is your ultimate source of inspiration and encouragement. When you make a mistake, just make a U-turn. Do you have a GPS device on your phone or in your car? When you make a wrong turn, the GPS doesn't call you an idiot. It just tells you where to make the next legal U-turn. If you pay attention to your mistakes, such as that you went too long between meals, didn't sleep, or failed to plan, these mistakes can be your best teachers.

Very soon you find yourself in a new place, where you have dramatically improved both your brain and your body.

God uses failure to educate us. Mistakes are simply learning experiences, and some things we learn only through failure. (So some of us are highly educated!)

Your setbacks can even reaffirm your faith. It may surprise you to know that admitting your hopelessness to God can be a statement of faith. King David said, "I believed in you, so I said, 'I am deeply troubled, LORD.' In my anxiety, I cried out to you" (Psalm 116:10–11 NLT).

David's frankness actually reveals a deep faith: First, he believed in God. Second, he believed God would listen to his prayer. Third, he believed God would let him say how he felt and would still love him.

Failure can also be motivational. A lot of times we change, not when we see the light, but when we feel the heat. When you fail, it's often an opportunity to take a different direction.

Regardless of your circumstances and how you feel, focus on who God is — his unchanging nature. Remind yourself what you know to be eternally true about God: He is good, he loves me, he is for me. He knows my struggles and my circumstances, and I know he has a good plan for my life.

TODAY'S STEPS

1. Ask a buddy how he or she makes U-turns and what helps them get back on track.
2. Journal about one setback, what you learned, and how you can make a U-turn and continue to make progress.

Energy Gains/ Energy Drains

Do not be anxious about anything, but in everything, by prayer and petition, with thanksgiving, present your requests to God. And the peace of God, which transcends all understanding, will guard your hearts and your minds in Christ Jesus. (Philippians 4:6-7)

Stress is a normal part of everyday life. Bad traffic, a big deadline, a fight at home — hundreds of things can stress us out. When the event passes, so does the stress, and we can breathe a big sigh of relief. With chronic stress, however, there is no relief. Chronic stress harms the brain. It constricts blood flow, which lowers overall brain function and prematurely ages your brain.

On a scale of 1 to 10, with 1 being absolutely no stress, and 10 being chronic stress, what is the current stress level in your life and why?

| 1 | 2 | 3 | 4 | 5 | 6 | 7 | 8 | 9 | 10 |

Many of us are losing energy because we have never taken the time to actually think about what is going on in our lives. Write a list of everything that gives you energy and everything that drains your energy. Include all persons, places, things, experiences, thoughts, feelings, and foods. What is it that is slowing you down? What brings you joy and helps you thrive? Each week resolve to let go of one thing that drains your energy and add one thing that gives you energy. Then incorporate the following stress-relieving activities into your life:

Pray on a regular basis. Decades of research have shown that prayer calms stress and enhances brain function.

Learn to delegate. Two of the greatest life skills you can learn are the art of delegation and the ability to say no.

Listen to soothing music. Listening to uplifting music that reminds you of God's truth can have a calming effect and reduce stress and anxiety.

Take a calming supplement. Some supplements may be helpful in soothing stress, but take these under the supervision of a healthcare professional. B vitamins, L-Theanine, and Gamma-aminobutyric acid (GABA) have calming effects. (*Note:* Pregnant women and nursing mothers should avoid L-theanine supplements.)

Exercise. When you are feeling low energy, exercise can be the thing to re-energize you. Keep going with the 40-day fitness plan.

TODAY'S STEPS

1. Identify your energy gains and drains.
2. Practice at least two to three ways to reduce your stress this week.

Meditate on God's Word

But they delight in the law of the LORD, meditating on it day and night. (Psalm 1:2 NLT)

No habit will help you in the spiritual dynamics of getting healthy more than meditating on and memorizing the Word of God. Jesus modelled this for us. Biblical meditation is not about emptying your mind but filling it with truth. It simply means to read a passage of Scripture, think about it, and repeat it to yourself. It's the first and most important step to memorizing Bible verses.

What do you need to change about the way you do your quiet time or structure your schedule so that you can fill your mind with the Word of God? Why not try thinking on God's character or his many names? (See pages 197 and 201 in *The Daniel Plan* book.)

As you bring your focus toward God, also bring it toward mindfulness in the other Daniel Plan Essentials. Be intentional about your food choices, your fitness, and your friends.

When you eat, do you intentionally sit, take your

time, chew your food, and remove all other distractions? There are two powerful benefits of mindful eating. First, you will eat less and enjoy your food more. Second, you will metabolize and burn food more efficiently. Study after study shows that when we eat unconsciously, we eat more. If you have a bigger plate, you will put more on it and eat more, so choose a smaller plate. As you savor each bite, you will eat less because you will enjoy your food more.

There are a few simple things you can do to eat more mindfully, get more pleasure from food, and design your environment. Then your mind will work on autopilot so you will naturally just do the right thing.

- Say a blessing of thanks before each meal.
- Always sit down and sit still.
- Eat from smaller plates.
- Stop and breathe before eating.
- Create a peaceful environment. Soft light, candles, quiet music, flowers.

Gratitude and prayer honor God and help focus your mind and bring you to the present moment. Start and end your day, your meals, and your exercise with both.

TODAY'S STEPS

1. Meditate on God's Word.
2. Use one mindful practice while eating.
3. Thank God before and after you exercise today.

Express Your Gratitude

Give thanks to the Lord, for He is good. (Psalm 107:1)

Where you bring your attention determines how you feel, and feeling grateful is a joyful place to be. This mindset builds your faith as you focus on the gifts God has given you. It helps you eat right as you focus on being grateful for the blessing of eating delicious, healthy food that serves your body. You realize how grateful you are for the renewed health of your body. Gratitude opens your heart to recognize how blessed you are by your family, friends, and community.

Modern medical research reveals that consistently focusing on your blessings and what you are grateful for each day has positive effects on your physical and mental health. A Yale University research study evaluated more than 2,000 veterans between the ages of 60 and 96 to assess which traits helped them age successfully. Gratitude and purpose were the most significant traits associated with successful aging. Your attitude matters.

Another study, from University of California-Davis, examined the effect of a grateful outlook on psychological and physical well-being. Participants were randomly assigned to one of three experimental conditions. They kept weekly or daily journals writing about hassles, gratitude, or neutral events. They also recorded their moods, coping behaviors, health behaviors, physical symptoms, and overall life appraisals. The grateful group exhibited the most heightened well-being.

Notice the connection Philippians 4:6-7 makes between gratitude and peace of mind: "Do not be anxious about anything, but in everything, by prayer and petition, *with thanksgiving,* present your requests to God. And the *peace of God,* which transcends all understanding, will guard your hearts and your minds in Christ Jesus." It's not enough just to present your requests to God. Do it with thanksgiving to enjoy peace of mind.

Every day write down three things you are grateful for. The act of writing down your gratitude enhances your brain. Then send a thank you note, post, tweet, or text to your Daniel Plan friends, acknowledging all the encouragement and support they have graciously offered you.

TODAY'S STEPS

1. Journal three things you are grateful for.
2. Send thanks to at least one friend.

Motion with Devotion

Prayer: God, I know you sent Jesus to die on the cross not just for my soul, but for my body. Thank you for another day where I get to honor you with my body. I intentionally choose to do that because I want to become Daniel Strong so I can live out the plan you've created for my life. I dedicate every movement to you.

The Daniel Plan integrates motion with devotion and brings back the fun and joy to your fitness and life. It makes sense, doesn't it? Sure, we can pop in the extreme fitness DVD or drag ourselves to the gym for a few weeks or months, but sooner or later, if we don't enjoy what we are doing, we are going to find a way out.

To help you experience motion and devotion throughout your busy day, here are a few ideas to help you whenever you find yourself sitting for long periods of time:

- Stretch your shoulders and arms, but close your eyes to worship God in silence.
- Squat up and down 5 to 10 times. With each repetition, thank God for the ability to move.

- Stretch your lower back and legs by slowly reaching down to touch your toes. Let this be a posture that expresses your devotion to God as you bow down to God's will in your life.
- Do 10 desk push-ups. Thank God for the use of your muscles and the health of your body.
- Go for a walking meeting instead of sitting in a conference room. Use this as a time of fellowship with others at work.
- Turn on some music and dance for a few minutes to your favorite song or worship music.
- Take a 2-minute recess. Use a hula hoop, jump rope, or Frisbee at work. Remind yourself that God loves when you smile and laugh and bring a cheerful and joyful heart to others.
- Take the stairs instead of the elevator. As you walk up, thank God for all he has done in your life, and share your worries with him. Tell him what you need.
- Stand when doing desk work. Let this be a reminder to you to stand for God in all you do.

Can you imagine the impact performing simple movements such as these, along with regular prayer, will have on your life?

TODAY'S STEPS

1. Incorporate prayerful movements throughout the day and during your exercise on the 40-Day Fitness Challenge.
2. Invite a friend to join you to do a new fitness movement/class.

Every Body Needs a Buddy

Two are better than one, because they have a good return for their labor: If either of them falls down, one can help the other up. (Ecclesiastes 4:9 – 10)

Part of becoming like Jesus and improving your health is to invite others to get healthy with you. The Bible says to put the interests of others above your own. God designed you to look out for others.

When you focus on others, you see that you are not alone and neither are they. Selflessly work for your friends' success as you would for your own. As you do so, you begin to truly believe that God can help you fulfill your goals because you see so clearly what he is doing in the lives of others.

Have you found a Daniel Plan buddy? For those of you who found a buddy day one, you've already experienced the power of friends. If you are doing The Daniel Plan through your church or on your own, it is vital to find a buddy at work or in your neighborhood who can do it with you. Getting healthy is a team sport, and being accountable to someone else and helping motivate and being motivated by a partner can double your success and make your changes stick.

Make a conscious effort to understand the health goals of your friends, family, or those in your Daniel Plan group. Then do something to encourage their health:

- Pray for your fellow group members on a regular basis.
- Send an email or write a card to one with the specific encouragement to reach his or her goals.
- Cook a meal and take extras to a friend or neighbor who may be living alone.
- Invite your Daniel Plan group for dinner.

TODAY'S STEPS

1. Extend an invitation to someone new to exercise together (a walk, hike, class).
2. Support a friend in changing his or her eating habits or cleaning out their pantry.

Pause, Celebrate, and Recalibrate

Congratulations! You have now finished 30 days of the 40-day experience. You are well on your way to making this your lifestyle. Celebrate the victories you have had along the way — every small step counts! How has your faith been impacted? How have your stress strategies helped you this far? Are you finding that daily meditation is helping you focus? Now that you have learned about the power of gratitude, have you integrated this into your daily routine?

Be sure to capture your thoughts in your journal so you can reflect on the progress you have made.

Embrace the fact that this is a journey, not a destination. Step by step you are making progress.

Looking ahead: You are on a roll! Your confidence is growing, and you are living a *healthstyle*. With all the healthy choices you've made this far, you have transformed in so many ways. We want to continue equipping you for success to run the race God has designed for you. Over the coming days you will further develop your skillset and accelerate your progress so you finish Daniel Strong.

Trust God Moment by Moment

Prayer: Lord, I need your power to help me every day, not just in my choices for better health, but also in my relationships, my work, and my faith. Breathe new life into my soul with your Holy Spirit, filling me with the power that comes only from you. In every moment, I choose to put my trust in you.

Where do you get the power to keep on going? You get it from God, by asking him to empower you and trusting in him moment by moment. God can make changes in your life that you have never dared to even dream of. He specializes in miracle makeovers. That is a power that you cannot find anywhere else.

This is the power you need to combat negative thought patterns, such as overgeneralization, blame, denial, thinking with your feelings, or predicting the future worst-case scenarios. (See page 36 of *The Daniel Plan Study Guide*.) God's Holy Spirit helps us break free from bad habits, compulsions, and addictions.

The more we allow God's Spirit to guide and empower us, the more he grows positive character qualities in our lives to replace our unhealthy habits.

You already know how important self-control is and the potential harm that can happen when you don't have it. But what most people don't know is that the secret of self-control is to allow ourselves to be Spirit-controlled.

His power comes when you practice biblical meditation and prayer. You can do this anywhere anytime. If you're at work, you can simply close the door to your office, sit in your chair, close your eyes, and pray. At home, you can sit on the edge of your bed and spend a couple of minutes calming your mind and focusing on God.

Relief from fear and worry is available in the moment you surrender and connect with God. You will find relief when you enter into his presence throughout the day. In a time of heightened stress, take time to pause, reflect, and refocus (even if it's in the car or the office).

Over and over in the Bible we are told "do not fear." In the moment you are fearful, reach out to God and trust that he is the ultimate remedy that eliminates fear. As a believer in Christ, delight in the fact that God's power is within your reach every moment of every day.

TODAY'S STEP

Put your trust in God's power rather than your
willpower.

Successfully Navigate Restaurants and Parties

Plenty of obstacles can come your way on this journey toward health. This is why planning is essential for your success. When it comes to meals and parties with friends, you have no doubt faced temptations. Turn your focus to the purpose of the event or celebration so you can adopt a new perspective. But also set yourself up for success by thinking ahead.

Part of life is going out and being with friends, going to events, eating at restaurants, and traveling. The good news is, you can eat almost anything occasionally and be fine — as long as it's real food, such as real pizza or French fries (not fast-food fries that have about 30 ingredients) or a piece of cake or cookies, and as long as you or someone you know made them from real ingredients.

Eating out is one of life's great pleasures. Our overall suggestion is to eat out less often and choose higher quality food when you do. When you go out, enjoy great food, and you will feel great too. Here are a few tips on how to eat well, feel well, and have fun eating out in restaurants and at parties while still following The Daniel Plan. (For additional ideas on eating out, check out pages 134 – 36 in *The Daniel Plan* book.)

- Skip the bread.
- Drink water, at least a glass or two, before you eat. You will likely eat less.
- Order two or three sides of veggies. Go crazy!
- Ask for extra virgin olive oil, vinegar, and fresh pepper for your salad instead of dressings.
- Choose foods associated with good words, such as roasted, broiled, baked, grilled, seared, steamed, sautéed.
- Skip the appetizer.
- Share entrées with a friend or companion.
- Never go to a party hungry.
- Bring your food. If you are going to a picnic, bring healthy choices to eat if there is nothing else worth eating.
- Start a trend with your friends. See who can find the best real food in your town.
- Say no to food pushers. These are people who say, "Come on, just have one bite" or "One can of soda can't hurt you." But have more respect for yourself and just say, "No thanks!"

TODAY'S STEPS

1. Plan ahead for meals that you will be eating out.
2. Bring healthy food options to parties.
3. Stay on track with your fitness routine and consider graduating to the next level.

Design Your Environment

Prayer: God, you establish my steps, and help me design my life with health in mind. I want to walk in your will and delight in your ways with full health, energy, and motivation.

Whether you work at home or in an office or travel a lot, designing your life -- knowing what to bring, where to shop, or where to eat in your immediate area — is a key to your success. Restock your emergency food packs and have a version for home, for work, for your car, for your travel bag. If you start to get hungry during the day, eat something. If you wait until you are starving, you will likely overeat.

At home, take stock of your kitchen again and make sure it has plenty of everyday foods — namely, an abundance of fresh non-starchy vegetables, lean protein, beans and legumes, whole grains, and seasonal fresh fruit and berries. Make your home a safe zone. Don't keep tempting junk, bad snacks, processed food, cookies, or cake in the house. If you want a treat or crave something sweet, have a piece of fruit or a piece of dark chocolate, or make something from scratch with real ingredients. You will eat less because you won't make it as often.

At work, think of a coworker who may want to collaborate with you to create a healthy work space.

God has given you a mission in life, and only you can fulfill it. We know you want to face your Savior at the end of your life and say, "I finished the race. I did what *you* put me on earth to do. I didn't get tired and worn out. I gave Jesus everything, including my physical health!"

Faith can virtually be regarded as a verb. It is active and not passive. Decision making is a faith-building activity. Use your muscles of faith to build your physical muscles. What are some of the best choices you made yesterday or today?

One Daniel Plan participant named Alonso dedicates the food he eats to God's purposes. He knows that change is his choice. His health journey has fueled new beliefs about God. He finds himself thinking differently: "If God can do this in my life (something I never thought possible), what else can he do?"

TODAY'S STEPS

1. Design your home and workspace to reflect healthy choices.
2. Journal about some of the best choices you've made that have built your health and your faith.

Mindset Matters

Finally, brothers and sisters, whatever is true, whatever is noble, whatever is right, whatever is pure, whatever is lovely, whatever is admirable — if anything is excellent or praiseworthy — think about such things. (Philippians 4:8)

Breathing is one of the few functions of your body that you do automatically — but it can also be done mindfully. When you remember to breathe deeply, you can actually calm your body and mind. By slowing your breathing, you can lower your heart rate and your stress level. Breathing is a powerful way to strengthen your body.

Mindful breathing reminds us to slow down and think about our choices, whether that concerns our faith, our food, our fitness, or our focus. For example, when we take a few deep breaths before we eat, we approach our eating more consciously. We eat less and enjoy it more. Here are a few other simple things you can do to be more mindful today:

- Chew each bite multiple times. You will improve digestion of your food and your enjoyment of it.
- Don't reward exercise by thinking, *I just walked 3 miles, so I can have a [fill in the blank].* Exercise is its own reward. Plus, if you have one 20-ounce soda, you have to walk 4.5 miles to burn it off. If you eat one super-size meal, you have to run 4 miles a day for one week to burn off that one meal. You can't exercise your way out of a bad diet.
- Don't shop hungry. If you are hungry when you shop, you are likely to buy more junk, quick snacks, processed foods, and fewer fruits and veggies.
- Buy in bulk, but then put food into small bags or containers. We tend to finish whatever size we start.

Today, take some time to breathe slowly and deeply. Regularly, repeatedly set aside time to quiet yourself and refocus your thoughts on the greatness and power of God. God can breathe new life into you and your efforts to become healthier.

TODAY'S STEPS

1. Incorporate deep breathing into your daily quiet time, before you eat, and before or after you exercise.
2. Reflect on the motivation that has brought you this far.
3. Incorporate a few mindful eating habits into your meals today.

Turn Ordinary Moments into Special Moments

Sitting down to eat a meal together is a great time to learn how everyone is doing. Whether you are eating with friends or sitting down to a family supper during the week, mealtimes help people stay connected. With demanding schedules and a multitude of activities, it's easy to see why eating together can often get derailed. But shared meals are a practice you will want to preserve. Consider a meal a date with your loved ones, a reservation that reveals how much you care.

Take time at the table for everyone to share about what's happening at school or work and talk about upcoming events. One approach that gets things started is called "highs and lows." Each person talks about a high point and a low point of the day or week. Letting each person open up in this way often leads to deeper conversations. Then go around the table and affirm each other. You'll be surprised how much you learn during just one meal!

Once a week or month, set the table for a party

to celebrate milestones and special achievements. Designate a special plate or table decorations for the occasion. When you stop to think about it, there is always something to celebrate besides birthdays, graduations, or anniversaries. Recognize an accomplishment at work or school, a deadline that was met, a new skill, an answered prayer, or a new friend. Celebrating together is a joy generator.

Take the leap. Set a schedule and send out the invitation. You'll wonder why you didn't do it sooner. It's a healthy way to nurture the ones you love. At some point, take it a step further and invite others to join your family, perhaps a friend who lives alone, a neighbor who has recently divorced, or anyone who could use some loving care. Open your door and your heart to share your meals and moments around the table. You will likely be inspired to make it an ongoing tradition.

> *Prayer: Lord, bless everyone who sits at my table. May they see your light and life radiating from me (and my family). Use me as an example of health that comes from relying on your power to change.*

TODAY'S STEPS
1. Make meals a family or neighborhood affair.
2. Plan a Daniel Plan potluck with your friends or family or at work.

Winning in the Kitchen

Every good and perfect gift is from above, coming down from the Father of the heavenly lights, who does not change like shifting shadows. (James 1:17)

Cooking is one of those acts that we have been doing for thousands of years. Ritual, tradition, and connection around food are part of every culture. Cooking is the most important food skill you have to create a rich, abundant healthy life. And cooking at home can be faster and cheaper than eating out.

In the time it takes to cook most packaged foods, you can make yourself a simple, delicious, healthy meal from real ingredients. You just have to have them in the kitchen ready to go.

If you are new to cooking from scratch, start with simple meals. Use just a few ingredients. Once you find a few quick, simple dinners or lunches that you and your family like, keep the ingredients in your fridge or freezer so that you are never stuck. Use the 40-day core meal plan in chapter 10 of *The Daniel Plan* book to get started.

To succeed in the kitchen:

- Get the right equipment. A few sharp knives will last a lifetime and make easy work of chopping and cutting vegetables. Good pans are easier to use and create better results.
- Learn basic cooking skills. You can take a class, but today you can learn almost any basic cooking skill online. Check out our Daniel Plan Chefs at *goo.gl/rntspb*.
- Prepare well. If you can read, you can cook! Getting all the ingredients ready, even measured, before you start to cook makes quick work of any meal. Read the recipe carefully. Check out *danielplan.com* for new recipe ideas.
- Know when it's done. The hardest part of cooking is learning when something is done. The vegetables should still be crisp, not soggy and limp. Overcooked chicken, meat, or fish is chewy and tough. You want to cook it until the pink is just gone. Fish is ready when it starts to flake apart when touched. Red meats should be cooked medium rare or medium.

Make your kitchen fun. Put on uplifting music, listen to podcasts of your favorite show, and invite family members and friends to share the preparation and cooking. If you have fun in the kitchen, you won't be afraid to get in there and cook more often.

TODAY'S STEPS

1. Cook at home.
2. Try a new recipe.

Try Something New

O Lord, what a variety of things you have made! In wisdom you have made them all. The earth is full of your creatures. (Psalm 104:24 NLT)

Look around, and you will see that God loves variety. He created people in different shapes and sizes. There are all kinds of trees and plants and so many choices of food we can eat. We even have choices within choices. For example, there are more than 7,500 varieties of apples.

God knows we need change and variety, and that includes our exercise routine. If your routine falls into a rut, exercise becomes less effective, and boredom (or even burnout) can creep in. That's why mixing it up can add new life to your fitness experience. You might get creative with your cardio exercise and wacky with your weight training.

What can keep you from getting bored? Driving a different route to work, trying a new kind of food, learning a new skill, or even meeting new people can help your brain and body stay healthy and active. Learn new ways to incorporate superfoods into your diet: avocado, broccoli, cacao, chia seed, flax seed, and kale just for starters. (For a more detailed list, check out the superfoods list in *The Daniel Plan Cookbook* on pages 35 – 39.) Or challenge your muscles to do a little bit more than you did yesterday. Mix it up, by increasing the number of reps, sets, or duration of exercise you perform. (See pages 180 – 83 of *The Daniel Plan* book for ideas.)

How about laughing more? There is a growing body of scientific literature suggesting that laughter counteracts stress and is good for the immune system. It's no joke! Laughter lowers the flow of dangerous stress hormones. Laughter also eases digestion and soothes stomach aches, a common symptom of chronic stress. Plus, a good rollicking chuckle increases the release of endorphins, which make you feel better and more relaxed. The average child laughs hundreds of times a day; the average adult laughs only a dozen times a day. Inject more humor into your everyday life.

Whatever new idea you choose to try, changing your routine will boost your fitness, sharpen your focus, and have you feeling a little bit lighter.

TODAY'S STEPS

1. When you exercise today, try a different activity from the options in the fitness plan.
2. Cook something new for dinner.
3. Read a funny book, watch a comedy, or share a funny story with someone else.

Rest in Him

You will keep in perfect peace those whose minds are steadfast, because they trust in you. (Isaiah 26:3)

As you work to renew your mind, stress will undoubtedly try to pull you away from your goals. The problems of everyday life often tempt us to make unhealthy choices out of convenience or as a temporary fix for handling stress. But the truth is, problems will follow you the rest of your life. If you're waiting to deal with stress until you make it to a new stage in your life, you will be waiting a long time!

Stress robs us of God's peace and clarity. We get stressed out when we focus on our own limited resources instead of focusing on the unlimited resources available through our heavenly Father. When we choose to focus on God, he strengthens us with his perfect peace. He helps us to stay balanced, focused, and strong. Focus on the fact that God is big enough to get you through any challenges you face.

Think about your morning and evening routines. Do you find yourself working on your laptop, or just sending off a few emails right before bed?

Are you completely rushed as you head out the door first thing in the morning? Small changes to your morning and evening routine can be simple, lessening your stress and helping you feel more rested. Try something like deciding you won't start working until you've gone for a walk and eaten a healthy breakfast, or won't end your day without prayer or an inspirational reading. Healthy boundaries like those will remind you that you are in control of your choices — and you will then be inspired to make healthier choices throughout the day.

One important truth to remember: God has given you the power to change your life, to set new patterns and reactions. Your daily choices, with God's limitless power, done with a community of friends, can help you launch each day with intention and purpose.

TODAY'S STEPS

1. Plan a day off with your friends.
2. Open your journal and write down what causes you the greatest stress, and ask God for help to relieve it.

Nothing Is Impossible with God

Now all glory to God, who is able, through his mighty power at work within us, to accomplish infinitely more than we might ask or think. (Ephesians 3:20 NLT)

God understands you better than you understand yourself. God knows what makes you tick — he knows what energizes you, what fatigues you, what makes you sick, and what makes you operate at your best. Doesn't it make sense to trust him to help you continue this journey toward long-term health?

The prophet Daniel didn't simply choose to eat healthier; he made that choice based on his faith, with a clear focus and the support of his friends. So it's no wonder that he was in better shape and health than the others in the king's court.

The powerful synergy of the Essentials — Faith, Food, Fitness, Focus, and Friends — combined with the support of friends brings you more than any one essential alone. None of them is less important than another. And each supports the others: When you feel weak in one essential, making positive change in the others restores your hope. As you move toward making the principles within all five a part of your daily lifestyle, you will have the strength to create change, sustain it, and maintain your motivation. Old refrains get rewritten, new stories are revealed, and life becomes an adventure powered by faith, hope, and love.

Now that you have established your Daniel Plan lifestyle, what goals are you considering to establish moving forward? Consider challenging yourself to a new level of fitness or sign up for a race or a new fitness activity. Share your success with someone you care about, and introduce them to your favorite healthy recipes. Ask God to inspire you toward even deeper faith and sharper focus. Pray about how God wants to use you to help others get healthy.

Invite people to join you on this journey. Enjoy the milestones God weaves in as he writes your story. Celebrate your successes. Share your struggles. Make a U-turn when necessary. Reframe failures as guideposts that serve you, not derail you. Get in community and live there, welcoming God's power into everything. This is the secret sauce of The Daniel Plan: getting healthy together, God's way and with God's power.

What is impossible from a human standpoint is easy to God. With God, today's impossibility is tomorrow's miracle. Are you ready for one?

TODAY'S STEPS

1. Start thinking about goals for the next 40 days.
2. Share your success with a friend.
3. Draw on God's limitless power to challenge your Faith, Food, Fitness, Focus, and Friends to a new level.

Better Together

*So it is with Christ's body. We are many parts of one body,
and we all belong to each other. (Romans 12:5 NLT)*

Our greatest desire is that you would embrace
The Daniel Plan and the five Essentials, inviting
health into every area of your life. Choose to believe
that all things are possible with God. Be kind to yourself, and trust him. Make God's Word a daily part of
your life, and his truths and promises will restore anything that's broken; his love will propel you into a new
way of thinking, a healthy approach to each day.

If you want to have lasting change in your life,
then you must fill your life with love. That's why
The Daniel Plan success depends on having friends
to walk beside you — because love is the only thing
that can change the unchangeable. It's the most powerful force in the world. Love invigorates, revitalizes,
and renews.

Love is the most irresistible force in the universe
because God is love. And that love is available and
accessible to every human being. We don't need to
earn it, only embrace it. The Bible doesn't say God

has love; it says he *is* love. Love is the core of his very nature. God's love heals what cannot otherwise be healed. God's love uplifts. It strengthens.

God designed us to grow spiritually within a supportive community. The same is true if we want to grow healthier.

When you connect with a loving community of friends, you will be better able to cope with things like fatigue, fear, frustration, and failure. You will be better able to handle depression and despair and, most important, not have to walk through them alone.

Community, when you embrace it, doesn't just help you succeed in your goals. It can bring you joy. Through deep relationships with others, you get to live in the love that God wants to give you. When you are surrounded by others who are just as committed to loving their neighbor as you are, then guess what: You're the recipient of that love as well as a giver of it.

As 1 John 4:12 says, "No one has ever seen God; but if we love one another, God lives in us and his love is made complete in us."

TODAY'S STEPS

1. Stay connected. Get social. Join us on your favorite social media venue. With whom can you share the information you have learned?

2. Take the Five Essentials Survey again. Go to
   danielplan.com/start and click on the link for
   "Essentials Survey."
3. Recheck your health numbers.

This Is Not the End

Here's the great news: This is just the beginning! This guide is designed to *launch* you on your journey to health. During these 40 days we have equipped you with spiritual inspiration and the basics of the five Essentials. The momentum from taking your early small steps is starting to take hold.

Celebrate your accomplishments, and express gratitude to God for his amazing work in you! Take some time to celebrate what you have accomplished. Grab your journal and write down answers to a few questions: What lasting changes have you made? How many pounds or inches have you lost? How, specifically, has your health improved — things such as lower blood pressure, reduced or eliminated medications, spiritual renewal, etc.?

Now that you have completed your 40-day journey, we encourage you to continue. Perhaps think of it as another continuing 40-day journey. As you keep building daily healthy practices, you are building momentum and making changes that will serve you for the long haul.

Where are you going from here? Now that you

have created your very own Daniel Plan lifestyle, what do you want to accomplish in the next 40 days? What one next step do you need to take in order to keep on running the race set before you? What do you need to embrace or reject? Perhaps your next step is to lead a Daniel Plan group. Visit *danielplan.com/tools* for next steps.

As you have learned, tracking your progress is key to sustaining change. Here are more practical next steps to choose from as you continue your journey to a healthier life!

Continue journaling: Get a new blank journal or create your own.

Sign up for our weekly newsletter: Sign up at *danielplan.com* to receive our weekly recipes, practical resources, everyday encouragement, biblical inspiration, fitness tips, and more.

Create new SMART goals in faith: Now that you have experienced the thrill of achieving your goals, it's time to take your health to a new level — think big!

Share The Daniel Plan: Now that you have a taste of everything The Daniel Plan has to offer, why not share it with a friend, coworker, or neighbor? Tell your faith community about it. Give the gift of health today.

Write us and share your story: *info@danielplan.com.*

The Daniel Plan

40 Days to a Healthier Life

Rick Warren D. MIN.,
Daniel Amen M.D.,
Mark Hyman M.D.

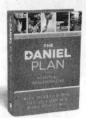

The Daniel Plan: 40 Days to a Healthier Life by Rick Warren, Dr. Daniel Amen, and Dr. Mark Hyman is an innovative approach to achieving a healthy lifestyle where people get better together by optimizing their health in the key areas of faith, food, fitness, focus and friends. Within these five key life areas, readers are offered a multitude of resources and the foundation to get healthy. Ultimately, *The Daniel Plan* is about abundance, not deprivation, and this is why the plan is both transformational and sustainable. *The Daniel Plan* teaches simple ways to incorporate healthy choices into your current lifestyle, while encouraging you to rely on God's power through biblical principles. Readers are encouraged to do The Daniel Plan with another person or a group to accelerate their results and enjoy a built-in support system. Readers are offered cutting-edge, real-world applications that are easy to implement and create tangible results.

Available in stores and online!

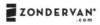